Automatic Athlete

Sports Specific Training System

Football

Leo Costa Jr.

Table of Contents

Introduction

Automatic Athlete Training System: The Product

Chapter 1

The Era of Specialization

Chapter 2

The Three Training Areas

Chapter 3

The Four Training Components

Chapter 4

Training Styles

Chapter 5

Training Techniques and Principles

Chapter 6

Training Phases/ Duration/ Repetition Ranges/ Rest Periods

Chapter 7

MCT™ Weights

Chapter 8

MCT™ Cardio

Chapter 9

MCT™ Diet and Nutrition

Automatic Athlete Training System

Introduction

12 years ago I took a trip to Bulgaria that changed my life forever. I was one of 26 Americans invited to study, train, and learn the cutting edge training methodologies of the Bulgarian Weight Lifting Team.

In a span of nine years, the Bulgarians had become the dominant powerhouse in Olympic weight lifting. This was an incredible feat considering that they were a very small country, not to mention, they essentially dethroned Russia who had always been number one in Olympic weight lifting.

Everyone in Europe wanted to know how and what training secrets the Bulgarians has stumbled upon to make them so dominant. I felt lucky that I was perhaps going to be privy to some of their secrets.

They were very creative and always thinking outside the box. They sometimes tried unorthodox training methodologies just to see if they would work, which in many cases, they did.

What I learned most from that incredible experience was to set specific goals, it is crucial to be creative and constantly thinking about attaining the goal.

If an athlete is trying to be as strong as possible, then his training and nutrition should reflect that. The same strategy would apply if more endurance or explosive power was the goal. It's that straight forward and simple.

That Bulgarian trip was directly responsible for my inspiratior to create a revolutionary exercise and nutrition training system and inventing the technology called **Micro Circuit Training™, which synergistically manipulates the three critical elements responsible for changing the body known as the three training areas.**

When I first started working as a personal trainer, my target clientele were people who were interested in getting into the best shape of their lives. Micro Circuit Training™ worked great because produced results quickly and efficiently.

After learning what I had in Bulgaria, about training and nutrition, I wanted to expand and start training athletes specifically for their sport. I was able to incorporate Micro Circuit Training™ int a very unique **sports specific training program** which manipulates the most critical elements that are responsible for developing the fu potential of the athlete, both physically and mentally. Micro Circuit Training™ technology takes away all guess-work on how athletes should go about reaching their full athletic potential efficiently.

Automatic Athlete Training System

The Product

Micro Circuit Training™ is definitely a life changing technology, and will impact athletes by changing how they look, feel, and perform automatically. This is how the product name (Automatic Athlete) evolved. Automatic Athlete is so efficient: an athlete can go about reaching their full athletic potential in as little as four hours per week. It doesn't get any more automatic than that.

Automatic Athlete is unique because it manipulates the most critical elements which are responsible for changing the body and implements a complete exercise and nutrition strategy. In addition, there is a psychological evaluation aspect which will determine how the athlete is hard wired.

Athletes must be both physically and mentally tough in order to efficiently compete in today's competitive sports arenas. Automatic Athlete and Micro Circuit Training™ will, without a doubt, **create the competitive edge.**

This means designing a sports specific training program, which takes advantage of the critical elements that change the mind and body in the most efficient way and create a process for the athlete that always works.

There are the primary training components known as the thre training areas which are weight training, cardio conditioning, and nutrition. However, it goes beyond the three training areas. It is crucial to manipulate the training phases utilizing the well establishe laws of adaptation. **This complete sport specific training progra** automatically incorporates this manipulation within the training phases.

It's important to have a sport specific training program that has structure but doesn't kill the variety. Within the program, creativity and challenges are built into the structure ensuring progress and results.

Automatic Athlete takes absolutely all of the guesswork out every part of the training program. The athlete can be confident th they are on the right training program.

The design of Automatic Athlete makes it virtually impossible for the body to ever hit plateaus. It is a sport specific training program that will change the stimuli automatically throughout a workout program according to the athlete's progress.

Easy, Simple, and Flexible Implementation

Automatic Athlete is easy to implement and flexible. It is typically a four day per week workout, Monday, Tuesday, Thursday, and Friday. The four days however, can be changed over a seven day period; as long as there is a one day's rest after two consecutive training sessions.

A different daily workout regime will be followed and will always include and manipulate all of the critical training elements. The training sessions last one hour; 30 minutes of weight training and 30 minutes of cardio. The weight training. Sessions are to be performed first.

And Finally

The information, knowledge, and results athletes will receive and gain from Automatic Athlete and the invention of MCT™ will be powerful and life changing. The techniques, training philosophy and design of this unique system have been tried and tested by myself on thousands of athletes that I have personally trained over the last 20 years. They always produce results.

It should also be known that there will always be athletes who will have special needs and want to take their athletic ability to an even higher level. For those individuals, we recommend subscribing to our very personal online Automatic Athlete Training System.

The online personal training program will utilize all of the same principles and technology of MCT™, while being even more specific to the athlete. The online personal training program has been set up in such a way that the athlete. The program has been set up in such a way that the athletes will truly feel like they have their own personal trainer working with them.

The beauty and benefit of this will be that athletes will pay a fraction of the cost compared to if they hired a full time trainer. On top of that, we are so confident of the results we will get, we are offering a money back guarantee.

I am very excited for you and look forward to hearing about the results you obtain.

Leo Costa

Chapter 1

The Era of Specialization

The Effects Upon a Training Program

Sports have changed dramatically in the last 30 years. One of the biggest changes is that athletes are now being asked to *specialize* more.

Back in the old days, football players used to play offense and defense. In baseball, pitchers used to throw entire games. It was common to be a multiple sport athlete and play in as many as three sports while still being competitive. That is not true today.

Athletes are not only being asked to specialize in one sport, but in one position in that sport. This is how specialized sports have come to be.

Since today's coaches new always looking for the competitive edge, it's extremely important that both coaches and athletes know specifically what needs to be done when implementing a sport specific training program. Specificity is key.

Athletes must be developed from the ground up - with specific goals in mind.

It All Starts with the Three Training Areas

As important as it is for athletes to practice and refine their skills through repetition on the field or court, they're only going to be as good as their foundation of **endurance, strength,** and **power.** Developing these foundations Strats way before the athlete's practice or play.

An athlete's overall *training methodology* is what creates the competitive edge. If there's a downfall or shortcoming during competition, it has its roots in the lack of specific implementation of the **three training areas.**

Chapter 2

The Three Training Areas

There are three training areas in a sport specific training program all of which are critical in helping an athlete reach their full athletic potential.

1. Weight Training
2. Cardiovascular conditioning
3. Nutrition

All three training areas are necessary. Leaving even one of these areas out of an exercise program will compromise overall results.

The primary functions of weight training are to tone or build muscle as well as improve metabolic functioning along with enhancing the body's ability for quicker recovery from workouts.

The primary functions of cardiovascular conditioning are to burn fat, and to eliminate the lactic acid created from weight training sessions; this helps speed up recovery for upcoming workouts.

The primary functions of nutrition are energy sourcing the body with adequate fuel for high energy workouts, keeping it healthy, and helping the body recover from workouts, not to mention its function for promoting fat loss and muscle gain.

Chapter 3

The Four Training Components

1. **Individual's Fitness Level -** There are three levels of fitness; novice, intermediate, and advanced. This indicates the level of experience that the individual has with regard to diet and exercise.

2. **Exercise Selection -** Choosing the right exercises to perform throughout your training program makes the training experienc a greatly productive one every time. In order for the exercises t produce maximum results, training circuits have been predetermined with a wide variety of exercises. The training circuits are designed to be specific to the five training phases which range from the novice to the advanced client.

3. **Repetition Ranges -** Repetition will vary and be specific tot he training phases, ranging from 6-20.

4. **Rest Periods -** Rest periods vary according to the client's abilit to do a volume of training as well as their efficiency of recovery.

Chapter 4

Training Styles

There are three applications of exercise training styles. These three styles can be applied simultaneously in the same workout session or in various combinations.

The three training styles are:

1. **Strict Style Training**
2. **Loose Style Training**
3. **Partial Style Training**

Strict style training can be used in various stages of any exercise program. For instance, it can be used when the individual is novice or advanced. Strict style training means keeping exercise form strict and doing a full range of motion - with the exercise tempo being at a moderate speed. Strict training is excellent for developing a foundation for the novice who needs to learn how to perform exercises correctly; as well as isolating a specific body part so that only that body part is being stimulated without the assistance of other muscle groups.

Loose style training utilizes a full range of motion during each exercise. Because it's used when lifting heavier weights, the rep tempo is more upbeat and aggressive. Momentum and other muscle groups assist in the exercise of the specific body part being trained - without the expense of being out of control.

Partial style training can be applied anywhere during a set and at any phase in training. Partials can be used in the beginning of a set as a pre-exhaust technique, as well as in the middle of a set, or even at the end of a set as a finishing technique. Partial training is an excellent way to push the muscle further than you could by only doing full range of motion exercises. Please note, that partial training should not be applied solely on its own.

Chapter 5

Training techniques and Principles

Combining Muscle Groups with Exercise

Combining multiple muscle groups with exercise is a very efficient and effective way to train in a 30-45 minute weight training session. The example of combining muscle groups would be as follows:

> From a seated position on a flat bench, holding dumbbells in a straight arm position, have the individual do dumbbell curls. The dumbbells are curled up to the shoulders, but instead of returning the dumbbells to the down position, which would complete the curl, the dumbbells are left at the shoulder position.
>
> At this point the individual will stand up from the bench, simulating a squat. As the individual stands up, they push the dumbbells overhead, doing a dumbbell shoulder press. After the press is complete, the dumbbells return back to the shoulders and at the same time, the individual is returning to a seated position. Just as the individual sits down, the dumbbells are returned to a down position completing the curl movement originally started.

This combination of muscle grouping and exercising is a way of training three different parts all at the same time (biceps, legs, and shoulders). This is an excellent way to thoroughly exhaust three different body parts all at once.

This is just an example of combining muscle groups in one exercise. There are many ways to be as creative as you want in terms of which muscle groups are combined with one another.

Finishing Techniques

A finishing technique would be considered a set extension technique used at the end of a set for any body part being trained. Again, the emphasis when training any body part is to make sure th the body part is thoroughly exhausted. Sometimes after regular exercises are performed, the body is still not thoroughly exhausted. Let's use the chest as an example. Bench press exercises along with a pec deck exercise were done, but let's say that for whatever reason, the chest muscles are still not fully exhausted. This is wher you can tweak a regular exercise by adding one more set to this body part by doing ULTRA HIGH REPS using the same exercises, like the bench press or the pec deck.

Always remember that even though rep ranges are established for each exercise, MUSCLES CAN'T READ - which means that after an exercise is performed and the rep range has been met, then this is the point when the finish technique can be applied.

Partials

Partials are another set extension technique used to tweak regular exercises. Partials can be used prior, during, or after any exercise being performed. Generally, when training any body part, full range of motion is used. Partials are an excellent way to tweak regular exercise in order to increase the intensity which will thoroughly exhaust the muscle.

Body Thru Space

Body thru space is yet another set extension technique that can be used to tweak regular exercises. *Body thru space* means using <u>body weight</u> to perform an exercise. This can be done without using any barbells, dumbbells, or any kind of weight training machines. One clear example is for the chest. Instead of doing a bench press, which is <u>not</u> a body thru space technique, the individual would do pushups or dips, which are *body thru space*.

An example of a *body thru space technique* for legs would be chain squats as opposed to leg extensions, which are not considered body thru space. The body thru space technique can be used before or after a regular exercise or even between regular exercises. This technique helps exhaust any muscle group much more efficiently.

Modify on the Fly

One of the worst things that can stifle results from an exercise program is **BOREDOM.** This often comes from doing the same workout for too long a period. An interesting fact to know is that the body will start adapting to any kind of routine in about 21 days. Staying on the same exercise routine for more than 3 weeks is death to getting results.

Variety is key to keeping the body off guard and never letting the muscle groups adjust to any kind of set routine. It keeps workouts fresh and the results coming on a consistent basis, which i the main objective.

The beauty of MCT™ principles and techniques are that the training applications are flexible, which an individual can modify to their workouts whenever needed.

Training through Injuries

At some point athletes will have to deal with injuries. In most cases, it is possible to train through and around injuries.

In fact, proper training can even promote healing and faster recovery. There are very few instances when an injured boc part needs complete rest. The example here would be if there was lower body injury, such as a pulled hamstring; the upper body can still be trained, as well as the rest of the lower body (except for the injured hamstring).

Again, in most cases, training an injured body part with very light training actually helps speed up recovery of the injury because new blood flow and improved oxygenation of the tissue.

The body has an amazing ability to adapt to its environment, whether it is in dealing with day-to-day stress or the environment of exercise stress. The body becomes its function, so over a period o time it can and will adapt to almost anything. Teaching the body to adapt to exercise stress, even injured body parts can have a very positive effect.

Life of a Rep

The life of a rep has to do with the quality of a set. It's not good enough just to do a bunch of reps during a set. The quality of the rep is extremely important. For example, if a set of 10 reps has been done, but only 4 of those 10 were quality, then 60% of that set was not performed to its highest potential.

The goal is to make sure every rep of every set counts, which means that every repetition being performed must be done with maximum efficiency. It's the quality - not quantity - that matters when performing reps for any body part. PERIOD!

Full vs. Partials

The equipment in a gym or studio should be thought of as tools that are used to thoroughly exhaust various muscle groups. This can be done by exercises that are performed through a full or partial range of motion. One is not necessarily better than the other. In fact, one without the other could minimize the benefit of how efficiently a muscle is trained.

The purpose of doing an exercise through a full range of motion is to thoroughly exhaust from where it attaches at its origination and insertion points. Another benefit of a full range exercise is that it promotes flexibility. However, only doing full range motions, DOES NOT thoroughly exhaust a muscle to its maximum potential. This is due to the fact that when a muscle is getting somewhat fatigued during a set, the tendency of momentum taking over or even stopping for a few seconds to rest before continuing the set allows the muscle just enough time to rest so it is not trained properly.

This is when doing partial repetitions can be applied, not only in the beginning of a full range exercise as a pre-exhaust technique, but also in the middle of the set , as well as at the end.

Individuals should use full range exercises as a foundation for training, and use partials as their secret weapon to thoroughly exhaust all muscle groups.

Acceleration and Deceleration

Accelerating and decelerating are techniques that can be used in weight training, cardio, and nutrition. Weight training, cardio, and nutrition (the three training areas) are three critical elements that need to be manipulated when an athlete is achieving their full athletic potential.

Acceleration and deceleration are excellent techniques to tak any one of the three training areas and shock the body for a temporary period of time. Sometimes through the course of training and nutrition, especially as an individual is getting into tip top shape, will be more difficult to get the body to respond to weight training, cardio, and nutrition.

Acceleration and deceleration can be applied simultaneously in the three training areas, as well as, applying in only one or two of the three training areas. It depends upon what the athlete needs.

Acceleration and deceleration, in regards to the three training areas and getting in top athletic shape, is like driving a car. Sometimes you need to go fast (acceleration) and sometimes you need to put on the brakes (deceleration). Manipulating the body to get into shape is no different.

Spotting

Spotting is extremely important for safety and performance. There is a right and wrong way for spotting. There are certain exercises that are more dangerous to perform. These require someone to be there who knows what to do in case the person performing the exercise prematurely fails or loses their balance.

A good spotter will potentially prevent a possible injury, as well as, help their partner do the exercise in a safe environment that can allow more reps. A good spotter should know where they should be in relation to the person doing the exercise. If a spotter is too close, they can be a distraction; if they are too far away, they are ineffective.

How to Manipulate a Diet

As an athlete is getting in better shape, there will be times when results can slow down or even come to a stop.

Temporarily shocking the body through diet manipulation is an excellent way to wake up a sluggish metabolism.

Increasing or decreasing calories should be used only at certain times and not as a mainstay of a nutritional program. This is strategy used to shock the body into results. Increasing or decreasing calories should be used no longer than 1-3 weeks at a time.

This is a great technique, but should be used wisely.

Chapter 6

Training Phases/ Duration/ Repetition Ranges/ Rest Periods

Automatic Athlete is a 16 week sports specific training program which consists of five training phases. Each phase is listed in the order and specific duration in which it should be implemented and completed.

Training Phases	Duration
1. Foundation Endurance	Two Weeks
2. Basic Strength Power	Five Weeks
3. Basic Body Balance/ Active Recovery Cardio	Two Weeks
4. Advanced Strength/ Power	Five Weeks
5. Advanced Body Balance/Active Recovery Cardio	Two Weeks

Explanation of Phases

Endurance - A level of muscle endurance must be developed in order to maximize the full athletic potential of all other training phases. One should implement as much variety as possible when choosing exercises.

Basic Strength/Power - Core exercises will be implemented and developed in this phase which will begin the development of a gooc technique and a solid base of strength and power.

Basic Body Balance/Active Recovery Cardio - A series of exercises will be implemented for the development of better athleti balance, as well as, a temporary recovery phase utilizing sport specific cardio conditioning techniques.

Advanced Strength/Power - Sport specific exercises will be developed to further develop the specific needs of the athlete for consistent peak performance on the field or court.

Advanced Body Balance/Active Recovery Cardio - A series of exercises will be implemented for the development of more advanced athletic balance, as well as, a temporary recovery phase utilizing sport specific cardio conditioning techniques.

Repetition Ranges/Rest Periods

Repetition ranges and rest periods will vary throughout the training program in accordance with each training phase.

Chapter 7

MCT™ Weights

Micro Circuit Training™ is a 30-45 minute workout, which experience has shown to be the optimum period for achieving maximum results. The strategy behind MCT™ is to train multiple body parts together.

MCT™ is a very effective and efficient way to do a lot of work in a short period of time. It is designed to be an up tempo workout program, which keeps an individual moving. Body parts are grouped in a circuit in such way for the individual to do a lot of exercise without having to spend very much time resting.

Generally MCT™ consists of three circuits. Three different exercises are done in each circuit. The same body part may be trained in the circuit, providing that different exercises are being performed. Each time a circuit is performed it is defined as a training round. There are three training rounds in each training session.

Repetitions may range from 6-20 and may go as high as 100. It all depends on the capability and fitness goals of the individual.

The sequence of exercises in each circuit can be modified at any moment, which is helpful when working in busy health clubs.

Because of the flexibility of MCT™ , there never is a problem with an individual not getting a great workout or with their training tempo getting interrupted or bogged down by other people working out in a crowded gym.

<u>Micro Circuit Training™ is designed to be a very efficient weight training program.</u>

In order for the body to change, it must be trained on the edge, without being over-trained. In other words, the body must be stressed to the point of fight or flight during the training session but without being overwhelmed.

MCT™ does this because the individual utilizing this training methodology is doing a lot of work in each one of the training circuits.

The body parts trained within each circuit are sequenced in a way that fatigues the muscle being trained thoroughly while allowing recovery for the other body parts that are a part of the training circuit.

The other advantage of MCT™ is that rest periods are kept to a minimum. A 30-45 minute MCT™ session can be used by individuals who are novices or highly trained athletes.

An example of a micro circuit of three exercises would be: Low Cable Row, Lat Pull Downs, and then Seated Chest Press. One could do them in any combination they wish. Notice that in the example of the circuit shown, there are two back exercises and one for the chest.

The way that a circuit should be executed is that the first exercise is performed for a certain amount of repetitions. Next, the second exercise is immediately performed with the repetitions designated, before moving on to the third exercise without stopping. After the third exercise is completed in the circuit, a rest period of approximately 30-45 seconds is taken.

In each micro circuit, the repetitions can be the same or completely different for each body part. MCT™ is designed to be extremely flexible and efficient. The most important thing an individual or trainer should always emphasize when weight training is that the body part being trained is thoroughly fatigued, but not over-trained.

In the Basic Strength/Power and Advanced Strength/Power training phases, a more conventional style of training is implemented. There will be a particular order of exercises and body parts are grouped.

Chapter 8

Active Recovery Cardio (ARC)

Active Recovery Cardio Training is a unique feature of the MCT™ program which is designed to help improve endurance, recovery, and eliminate body fat.

The body has natural cycles it transitions through as it's responding and adapting to diet and exercise. It is especially important with athletes that training is done at intense levels withou experiencing burnout.

This can be done, if an exercise program is implemented properly, an athlete can be in or near peak performing shape year round. This is accomplished by changing the training stimulus in a specific way.

Active Recovery Cardio (ARC) is a training component of Micro Circuit Training™ , and coincides with the weight training and nutrition components.

Throughout the sports specific training program cardio will b performed; mainly as a specific tool which benefits the athlete. It w be used as a short warm up prior to a weight training session or aft as a recovery to help eliminate the onset of muscle soreness. ARC will also be used to do interval training and eliminate unnecessary body fat.

ARC will play a key role throughout the sport specific training program to continue to help the athlete recover from workouts. It is a well known fact that recovering from training sessions is as important as the training sessions themselves.

Cardio conditioning for the football athlete will be broken down into four categories and implemented according to the specific needs of the athlete.

1. Warm Up
2. Endurance
3. Interval
4. Lactic Acid Flush

Explanation of Categories

Warm Up - Sometimes a ten minute cardio warmup prior to a weight training workout is necessary for the athlete to get the blood flowing as well as loosening up body parts that are sore or slightly injured.

Endurance - Develops muscle endurance, which increases the body's ability to perform more efficiently at higher levels and improves recovery time. Endurance training will also be implemented for the athlete that must drop body fat. Heart rate should be kept at 75% of max heart rate.

Interval - Interval training is an increase of speed of explosive bursts, which can last between 15 seconds to a minute, followed by a return to normal speed, and then repeated several times over a 20 minute training session. Interval training will significantly improve foot speed and quickness.

Lactic Acid Flush - Is used as a tool to help flush out lactic acid which builds up as a result of an intense workout. Lactic Acid Flush will speed up recovery in between weight training workouts. Lactic Acid Flush is to be done after weight training sessions.

The Aerobic Heart Rate Formula

The formula below shows how to arrive at an ideal heart range for burning body fat:

Step 1: 220 minus age equals maximum heart rate.

Step 2: Max heart Rate times 0.7 equals low end ideal heart rate to burn body fat.

Step 3: Max heart rate times 0.85 yields the high end ideal heart rate to burn body fat.

Cardio Training Schedule

Week 1

Category - Endurance

Action - 4 days per week, 30 minutes after each weight training session. Heart rate 75% of max. Walk, jog, or run is acceptable.

Week 2

Category - Endurance

Action - 4 days per week, 20 minutes after each weight training session. Heart rate 80% of max. Walk, jog, or run is acceptable.

Week 3 - 4 - 5

Category - Lactic Acid Flush

Action - 3 days per week, 10-15 minutes after each weight training session. Heart rate 70% of max. Walk, jog, or run is acceptable.

Week 6

Category - Interval

Action - 4 days per week. Cardio session lasts 15 minutes to 30 minutes. Sprint burst for 15 seconds with 2 minutes rest between each burst. Complete 6 bursts.

Week 7

Category - Interval

Action - 4 days per week. Cardio lasts 17 minutes 45 seconds. Sprint bursts for 15 seconds, with 2 minutes rest in between each burst. Complete 7 bursts.

Week 8

Category - Interval

Action - 3 days per week. Cardio lasts 20 minutes. Sprint bursts fo 15 seconds with 2 minutes rest between each burst. Complete 8 bursts.

Week 9

Category - Interval

Action - 3 days per week. Cardio lasts 22 minutes 15 seconds. Sprint bursts for 15 seconds with 2 minutes rest in between each burst. Complete 9 bursts.

Week 10

Category - Endurance

Action - 3 days per week. 30 minutes after each weight training session. Heart rate 80% of max. Walk, jog, or run is acceptable.

Week 11 - 12 -13

Category - Lactic Acid Flush

Action - 3 days per week. 10-15 minutes after each weight training session. Heart rate 70% of max. Walk, jog, or run is acceptable.

Week 14

Category - Interval

Action - 4 days per week. Cardio session lasts 15 to 30 minutes. Sprint burst for 15 seconds with 2 minutes rest between each burst. Complete 6 bursts.

Week 15

Category - Interval

Action - 3 days per week. Cardio lasts 9 minutes 45 seconds. Sprint burst for 15 seconds with 1 minute rest in between each burst. Complete 7 bursts.

Week 16

Category - Interval

Action - 3 days per week. Cardio lasts 13 minutes 50 seconds. Perform 1 sprint burst with 1 minute rest in between each burst. 3 sprint bursts with 45 seconds rest in between each burst. 3 sprint bursts with 30 seconds rest in between each burst. 1 burst with 2 minute rest in between each burst. Complete 11 bursts.

Chapter 9

MCT™ Diet and Nutriton

There is a tremendous amount of confusion in the diet and nutrition industry, especially when it comes to knowing what **type** o diet or nutrition program should be followed.

First it must be understood that our body functions and operates off of two metabolisms. Specifically one or the other.

1. Free Fatty Acid Metabolism
2. Glucose Metabolism

In order to determine which metabolism is dominant, a diet analysis must be performed on the individual by a doctor or dieticia If an individual is consuming on a daily basis, 30 grams of carbohydrates or less, the Free Fatty Acid Metabolism is dominant. If carbohydrate consumption is above 30 grams, the Glucose Metabolism is dominant.

The diet analysis will also serve as a tool to determine daily calorie consumption, which will be useful when determining which calorie category the individual should be put in.

Both metabolisms are effective and can be incorporated throughout MCT™. It is important to know that in order to maximiz results; only one type of diet should be followed at a time, which should be determined by the individual's physician or dietician.

MCT™ diet and nutrition is the third component of the three training areas, which are part of the MCT™ system. MCT™ diet and nutrition has been broken down into two metabolism categories: 1. Glucose Metabolism (GM) 2. Free Fatty Acid Metabolism (FFAM), which indicate the type of diet.

MCT™ diet and nutrition also has 3 specific calorie categories: 1. Weight loss 2. Weight Maintenance 3. Weight Gain. These are calorie ranges for males depending on their specific goal.

Below are the calorie breakdowns in the three categories for males

Weight Loss (calorie kickdown)	1500-1800 calories
Weight Maintenance	1800-2500 calories
Weight Gain (calorie kickup)	2500-3000 calories

Note

MCT™ diet and nutrition strategy is carefully designed to work in conjunction with MCT™ weight training and cardio. There are specific times throughout MCT™ diet and nutrition where calorie changes are being made in order to maximize results.

It is recommended for the individual to stay on one **type** of diet and **not** combine the two at one time. The type of diet can be changed throughout MCT™; however it is recommended to stay on one type of diet for two weeks before changing.

Diet and nutrition does not have to be complicated, and yet o the three training areas of MCT™, the diet and nutrition is the most difficult for individuals to follow through. There are many diets one can follow, so it's difficult and confusing for individuals to know where to start.

Our recommendation and strategy is to keep things simple y effective. There are simple things to remember that will always be true. All diets work to a degree. Not one diet on the market will be the sole answer, but some will work better than others.

Calories initially are the most important variable. It takes so many calories to maintain body weight, and so many to gain or lose weight. Another important thing to know about your diet is that the are recommended daily allowances with regard to how much prote carbs, and fat should be consumed. Consult a dietician or doctor t find out this information.

Knowing which diet to follow is a process, and there is a certain amount of trial and error to get it dialed in.

The strategy we suggest is simply this: Once a diet analysis completed, choose what your objective is, and pick the calorie category that matches your objective. As far as which type of diet follow, just pick one, any one, it does not matter. We suggest that you consult your doctor or dietician. Stay on the diet you choose f two weeks. If, after two weeks, there are no results, make a chang

The objective is to give the body a chance to respond to the type of diet you're following. Two weeks will be enough to make a properly informed decision.

You must know how to objectively measure results. There are two very simple things you can do: 1. Pay attention to how your clothes start fitting. Once you begin a diet, are they getting looser, fitting the same, or getting tighter? 2. Weigh yourself every Friday, first thing in the morning. These two things will give you good information pertaining to what you should do. It is also suggested to do a diet analysis every 3-4 weeks in order to maintain accountability. It's that simple! A diet needs to be user friendly and something that can be followed consistently.

Any time an individual makes changes to their diet, they should consult a physician or dietician.

Diet and Nutrition Schedule

Diet and nutrition is the third component of the three training areas, and must be implemented at specific times throughout MCT™. Below is the diet and nutrition schedule, which coordinates with MCT™ weight training and cardio conditioning.

Weeks 1 and 2 - During weeks 1 and 2 of MCT™, the emphasis should be on getting acclimated to weight training and cardio conditioning. However, during weeks 1 and 2, a 2 day food journal should be filled out and a diet analysis completed. By the end of week 2 the individual should know the results of their diet analysis.

Week 3 - Week 3 will be a calorie kick down week. If at week 3, the individual has not started to meet their fitness goals, a kick down in calories for the week would be implemented. At this point the individual will be put in the weight loss category.

Weeks 4 and 5 - On weeks 4 and 5, the individual will get a caloric kick up. They will be put in the weight maintenance category for 2 weeks.

Weeks 6 and 7 - On weeks 6 and 7, if the individual is still not meeting their fitness goals, a calorie kick down will be implemented. The individual will be put in the weight loss category.

Weeks 8 and 9 - On weeks 8 and 9, the individual will get a calorie kick up. They will be put in the weight maintenance category for 2 weeks.

Weeks 10, 11, and 12 - These three weeks will be the most intense in terms of calorie kick down, in part because of the length of time. The individual will be put in the weight loss category.

Explanation

The diet and nutrition schedule is designed to work in conjunction with the various training phases of MCT™. There are specific weeks where calorie kick downs are implemented in order to stimulate the metabolism for those individuals who need it.

If an individual is on schedule as far as their fitness goals are concerned, then it is not necessary to implement calorie kick downs on the designated weeks. The individual could stay in the weight maintenance category throughout the entire MCT™ program.

For those individuals interested in gaining weight, on the specific weeks designated for calorie kick downs, a calorie kick up would be implemented instead. The individual in this scenario would be put in the weight gain category and then return to weight maintenance.

MCT Football

Football is a sport which involves endurance, strength, and power. These three areas should be the main focus in the weight room for an off season football program. The MCT™ Football program focuses on these three areas to specifically condition the athlete for the fundamentals of football.

Endurance is often thought of as the cardiovascular conditio of an athlete. For instance, how far one can run without tiring or ho fast an athlete can recover. While these are also related to football, muscle endurance is our focus in the weight room.

Football is a physical sport, which involves pushing and pulling one's own body as well as others through space play after play, just being strong will not be enough in the 4th quarter. This is why it is so important that the athlete's muscles are not only conditioned to be strong, but to have endurance as well.

It is well known that you cannot have maximum gains in strength until the muscle is conditioned for endurance first. This means higher reps and volume at the beginning. Once the muscle conditioned for endurance, a true strength and power program can be implemented.

Endurance is the first training phase of MCT™ Football, whic lasts two weeks and emphasizes a full body endurance workout. This means that all of the lifts and movements are done for higher reps and volume.

Basic Strength/Power is the second training phase which lasts five weeks and emphasizes the good development of not only strength/power, but perfect form, technique, and execution of movements. Repetition ranges in this training phase will be lower and rest periods will increase.

Basic Body Balance/Active Recovery Cardio is the third training phase which lasts two weeks and emphasizes body awareness through dynamic, ballistic, and static movements; as well as the implementation of cardio conditioning techniques to help aide in full body recovery.

Advanced Strength/Power is the fourth training phase which lasts five weeks and emphasizes specific strength and power that is specific to the characteristics of the sport. Unlike in the second training phase (basic strength/power), a bigger variety of exercises will be implemented.

Advanced Body Balance/Active Recovery Cardio is the fifth and final training phase which lasts two weeks. This training phase is more intense and continues to challenge athletes in becoming more aware of how their bodies move through space, and also trains the body to recover more efficiently.

The MCT™ program has been specifically designed for football players to reach their full athletic potential, and be peak performers on the field. This has been accomplished by controlling and manipulating all of the elements of a sports specific training program.

Training Phases/Schedule

Endurance Training

Weeks 1-2

This is a three day per week workout. Any combination of 3 days of training is acceptable as long as there is a one day rest in between each workout.

There are three circuits to be performed each day. There are three training rounds performed in each circuit. All three training rounds must be performed in their entirety before moving on to the next circuit.

In order to add variety, there are A and B workouts listed in each circuit. This means if the exercise in the A list is being used and the gym is busy, or perhaps does not have the piece of equipment needed, then the B list can be used.

- Repetition ranges are to be kept between 10-20 for each trainin round and circuit.
- Rest periods are taken as needed between each training round.
- Abdominals are performed at the end once all of the circuits are completed.

Basic Strength/Power

Weeks 3-7

This is a 4 day per week workout. Combinations of strength and power exercises are performed. There should be two consecutive training days performed with a one day rest in between, before training two more consecutive days.

There is an order in which the exercises should be performed. By design there will be a certain amount of redundancy, in order to become more proficient at properly executing the strength and power moves.

There are five sets per body part being performed throughout the training phase. All sets must be performed in their entirety before moving on to the next body part.

- Repetition ranges are kept from 5-8 for each set.
- Rest periods can last up to 1 minute for each set.
- Abdominals are performed at the end of each workout session.

Basic Body Balance/Active Recovery Cardio (ARC)

Weeks 8-9

With respect to the body balance segment, there are three training circuits performed each day. There are three training rounds performed in their entirety before moving on to the next circuit.

There is an order in which the exercises should be performed. By design there will be a certain amount of redundancy, in order to become more proficient at properly executing the basic body balance movements.

Repetition ranges are kept between 10-15 for each training round and circuit.

- Rest periods are taken as needed between each training round.
- With respect to ARC, interval will be the training protocol.
- Abdominals are performed at the end once all circuits are completed.

Advanced Strength/Power

Weeks 10-14

This is a 4 day per week workout. Combinations of strength and power exercises are performed. There should be two consecutive training days performed followed by one day's rest in between, before two more consecutive training days.

There is an order in which the exercises should be performed. By design there will be a certain amount of redundancy, in order to become proficient at properly executing the strength and power moves.

There are 5 sets per body part being performed throughout the training phase. All sets must be performed in their entirety before moving on to the next body part.

- Repetition ranges are kept from 5-8 for each set.
- Rest periods can last up to 1 minute for each set.
- Abdominals are performed at the end of each workout session.

Advanced Body Balance/Active Recovery Cardio (ARC)

Weeks 15-16

With respect to the body balance segment, there are three training circuits performed each day. There are three training round performed in each circuit. All three training rounds must be performed in their entirety before moving on to the next circuit.

There is an order in which the exercises should be performed By design there will be a certain amount of redundancy, in order to become more proficient at properly executing the advanced body balance moves.

- Repetition ranges are kept between 10-15 for each training round and circuit.
- Rest periods are taken as needed between each training round.
- With respect to ARC, interval will be the training protocol.
- Abdominals are performed at the end once all of the circuits are completed.

Explanation

Endurance exercises are specifically designed to develop and increase muscle endurance and recovery to maximize the potential of the other three training phases.

Strength and power exercises are specifically different training applications. Strength exercises are specifically designed to make an athlete stronger and are to be executed in a deliberate and precise manner.

Power exercises are specifically designed to make an athlete more explosive, which also develops speed.

Body balance exercises are specifically designed to make an athlete more aware of how to control his or her body through dynamic, ballistic, and static movements.

Automatic Athlete

16 Week Workout

There are 3 exercise rounds performed in each circuit. All 3 rounds must be performed in their entirety before moving on to the next circuit.

Endurance Training Week 1

	Day 1	
	Circuit 1	
	Exercise	**Reps**
1a	Squats	**10-15**
1b	Smith Machine Bench Squats	**10-15**
2a	BB Chest Press	**10-15**
2b	DB Flat Chest Press	**10-15**
3a	Seated Calf Raise	**10-15**
3b	Close Grip BTS Bar Pushup	**10-15**
	Circuit 2	
4a	Lat Pull Down	**10-15**
4b	Assisted BTS Chinups	**10-15**
5a	Smith Seat Shoulder Press	**10-15**
5b	Stand DB Shoulder Press	**10-15**
6a	BB Stand Curl	**10-15**
6b	Cambered Bar Close Grip Stand	**10-15**
	Circuit 3	
7a	Lying Leg Curl	**10-15**
7b	Stand Smith Machine Dead Lift	**10-15**

	Day 2	
	Circuit 1	
	Exercise	**Reps**
1a	Leg Press	**10-15**
1b	Hack Squat	**10-15**
2a	Incline DB Fly	**10-15**
2b	Smith Machine Flat Bench	**10-15**
3a	DB Tri Kickback	**10-15**
3b	Stand Rope Triceps Pushdown	**10-15**
	Circuit 2	
4a	Low Cable Row	**10-15**
4b	DB One Arm Row	**10-15**
5a	DB Front Raise	**10-15**
5b	Stand Cambered Bar Front Raise	**10-15**
6a	Seated DB Curl	**10-15**
6b	Stand Rope Curl	**10-15**
	Circuit 3	
7a	DB Alt Squats	**10-15**
7b	Wide Stance Straddle DB Squat	**10-15**

	Day 3	
	Circuit 1	
	Exercise	**Reps**
1a	BTS Toe Raise	**10-1**
1b	Hyperextensions	**10-1**
2a	Cable Cross Over	**10-1**
2b	Incline Cable Cross Over	**10-1**
3a	Bench Dip	**10-1**
3b	Incline Rope Triceps Pushdown	**10-1**
	Circuit 2	
4a	Straight Arm Pulldown	**10-1**
4b	Close Grip Front Lat Pulldown	**10-1**
5a	DB Side Lateral Raises	**10-1**
5b	Stand Cambered Bar Upright Row	**10-1**
6a	Lying Leg Curl	**10-1**
6b	Standing Stick Goodmornings	**10-1**
	Circuit 3	
7a	Chain Squats	**10-**
7b	Smith Machine Stepups	**10-**

8a	Incline DB Chest Press	**10-15**
8b	Cable Cross Over	**10-15**
9a	Stand Triceps Pushdown	**10-15**
9b	Seated Triangle Triceps Extension	**10-15**
Abdominals 3 Supersets		
Bicycle Crunch		**50**
Flutter Kicks		**50**

8a	Pec Deck	**10-15**
8b	Incline Smith Machine Chest P	**10-15**
9a	Stand Triceps Extension	**10-15**
9b	Flat Close Grip Bench Press	**10-15**
Abdominals 3 Supersets		
Ball Crunch		**15-20**
Windmills		**15-20**

8a	Pushups	**10-15**
8b	DB Flat Bench	**10-15**
9a	DB Triceps Kickback	**10-15**
9b	Bent Over Triceps Rope Extension	**10-15**
Abdominals 3 Supersets		
Hanging Knee Raises		**20**
Kneel Cable Crunch		**20**

There are 3 exercise rounds performed in each circuit. All 3 rounds must be performed in their entirety before moving on to the next circuit.

Endurance Training Week 1

Day 1

	Exercise	Reps
	Circuit 1	
1a	BB Chest Press	**10-20**
1b	DB Flat Chest Press	**10-20**
2a	Seated Calf Raise	**10-20**
2b	Close Grip BTS Bar Pushup	**10-20**
3a	Squats	**10-20**
3b	Smith Machine Bench Squats	**10-20**
	Circuit 2	
4a	Smith Seat Shoulder Press	**10-20**
4b	Stand DB Shoulder Press	**10-20**
5a	BB Stand Curl	**10-20**
5b	Cambered Bar Stand CG Curl	**10-20**
6a	Lat Pulldown	**10-20**
6b	Assisted BTS Chinups	**10-20**
	Circuit 3	
7a	Incline DB Chest Press	**10-20**
7b	Cable Crossover	**10-20**
8a	Stand Triceps Pushdown	**10-20**
8b	Stand Triceps Pushdown	**10-20**
9a	Lying Leg Curl	**10-20**
9b	Stand Smith Machine Deadlift	**10-20**
Abdominals 3 Supersets		

Day 2

	Exercise	Reps
	Circuit 1	
1a	Incline DB Fly	**10-20**
1b	Smith Machine Flat Bench	**10-20**
2a	DB Tri Kickback	**10-20**
2b	Stand Rope Triceps Pushdown	**10-20**
3a	Leg Press	**10-20**
3b	Hack Squat	**10-20**
	Circuit 2	
4a	DB Front Raise	**10-20**
4b	Stand Cambered Bar Front Raise	**10-20**
5a	Seated DB Curl	**10-20**
5b	Stand Rope Curl	**10-20**
6a	Low Cable Row	**10-20**
6b	DB One Arm Row	**10-20**
	Circuit 3	
7a	Pec Deck	**10-20**
7b	Incline Smith Machine Chest Press	**10-20**
8a	Stand Triceps Extension	**10-20**
8b	Flat Close Grip Bench Press	**10-20**
9a	DB Alternating Lunges	**10-20**
9b	Wide Stance Straddle DB Squat	**10-20**
Abdominals 3 Supersets		

Day 3

	Exercise	Reps
	Circuit 1	
1a	Cable Crossover	**10-20**
1b	Incline Cable Crossover	**10-20**
2a	Bench Dip	**10-20**
2b	Incline Rope Triceps Pushdown	**10-20**
3a	Lying Leg Curl	**10-20**
3b	Hyperextensions	**10-20**
	Circuit 2	
4a	Side Lateral Raises	**10-20**
4b	Stand Cambered Bar Upright Row	**10-20**
5a	BTS Toe Raise	**10-20**
5b	Standing Stick Good Mornings	**10-20**
6a	Straight Arm Pulldown	**10-2**
6b	Close Grip Front Lat Pulldown	**10-2**
	Circuit 3	
7a	Pushups	**10-2**
7b	DB Flat Bench	**10-2**
8a	DB Triceps Kickbacks	**10-2**
8b	Bent Over Triceps Rope Extension	**10-2**
9a	Chain Squats	**10-2**
9b	DB Alternating Lunges	**10-2**
Abdominals 3 Supersets		

Bicycle Crunch	50	Ball Crunch	15-20	Hanging Knee Raises	20
Flutter Kicks	50	Windmills	15-20	Kneel Cable Crunch	20

Explanation
Repetition Sets and Rest for
Strength, Power, Body Balance

Repetitions (Reps), Sets, and Rest are three very important components when performing a workout. Repetitions are the number of times in which each exercises movement is performed. If the workout requests 6 repetitions, it means the individual movement is to be done 6 times before resting.

There are also sections of the workout that request Max Repetition. This means that the exercise or movement should be performed as many times as possible without sacrificing form/ technique and without rest.

Sets refer to the number of times each exercise is performed at the given amount of repetitions. For instance, if the workout calls for 6 repetitions and 5 sets, the given exercise will be for 6 repetitions 5 times. This means a total of 30 repetitions will be done at 6 repetitions at a time.

Rest refers to the amount of time taken between each set. If the rest period calls for 1 minute, then 1 minute should be taken for rest before starting right after the last repetition of the set. If the rest period calls for Full Recovery this means that after the last repetition is performed you should be fully rested before performing the next set of repetitions.

Minimum Recovery is exactly the opposite; when the workou calls for this it simple means that after the set is performed you should perform the next set as soon as you can.

Abdominal Explanation

Pyramid Abs - These are Crunches, Leg Lifts, and V Ups. Yo are to perform each exercise in the order given. The repetitions are little different here because the amount of reps change as you complete each set. For instance, the repetitions for Pyramid Abs in week 3 start with 20 reps and work down to 5 for the last set.

This means that you are to perform Crunches, Leg Lifts, and Ups for 20 reps each for the first set, then descend to 15 reps the second set, 10 the third, and finally 5 reps for the fourth set.

BB Abs - Crunches/Leg Lifts - These are simply crunches ar leg lifts performed while holding the 45 pound barbell at arm's leng over your chest.

Basic Strength/Power

Weeks 3-7

Week 3

Day 1 Upper Body

Exercise	Repetitions	Sets	Rest
Flat Bench BB	6	5	1 minute
Incline bench BB	6	5	1 minute
Clap Pushup	6	5	1 minute
Pull Up	6	5	1 minute
BB Row	6	5	1 minute
Pushup	Max	3	Full Recovery
Inverted Row	Max	3	Full Recovery
Pyramid Abs Crunch/Leg Lift/V Up	20 descending to 5	4	Minimum Recovery

Week 3

Day 2 Lower Body

Exercise	Repetitions	Sets	Rest
Power Clean	6	5	1 minute
Hang Clean	6	5	1 minute
Snatch	6	5	1 minute
Back Squat	6	5	1 minute
Front Squat	6	5	1 minute
Military Press	6	5	1 minute
BB Abs Crunch/Leg Lift	20Superset	3	Full Recovery

Week 3

Day 3 Upper Body

Exercise	Repetitions	Sets	Rest
Flat Bench BB	6	5	1 minute
Incline bench BB	6	5	1 minute
Clap Pushup	6	5	1 minute
Pull Up	6	5	1 minute
BB Row	6	5	1 minute
Pushup	Max	3	Full Recovery
Inverted Row	Max	3	Full Recovery
Pyramid Abs Crunch/Leg Lift/V Up	20 descending to 5	4	Minimum Recover

Week 3

Day 4 Lower Body

Exercise	Repetitions	Sets	Rest
Power Clean	6	5	1 minute
Hang Clean	6	5	1 minute
Snatch	6	5	1 minute
Back Squat	6	5	1 minute
Front Squat	6	5	1 minute
Military Press	6	5	1 minute
BB Abs Crunch/Leg Lift	20 Superset	3	Full Recovery

Week 4

Day 1 Upper Body

Exercise	Repetitions	Sets	Rest
Flat Bench BB	7	5	1 minute
Incline bench BB	7	5	1 minute
Clap Pushup	7	5	1 minute
Pull Up	7	5	1 minute
BB Row	7	5	1 minute
Pushup	Max	3	Full Recovery
Inverted Row	Max	3	Full Recovery
Pyramid Abs Crunch/Leg Lift/V Up	20 descending to 5	4	Minimum Recovery

Week 4

Day 2 Lower Body

Exercise	Repetitions	Sets	Rest
Power Clean	7	5	1 minute
Hang Clean	7	5	1 minute
Snatch	7	5	1 minute
Back Squat	7	5	1 minute
Front Squat	7	5	1 minute
Military Press	7	5	1 minute
BB Abs Crunch/Leg Lift	20/Superset	3	Full Recovery

Week 4

Day 3 Upper Body

Exercise	Repetitions	Sets	Rest
Flat Bench BB	7	5	1 minute
Incline bench BB	7	5	1 minute
Clap Pushup	7	5	1 minute
Pull Up	7	5	1 minute
BB Row	7	5	1 minute
Pushup	Max	3	Full Recovery
Inverted Row	Max	3	Full Recovery
Pyramid Abs Crunch/Leg Lift/V Up	20 descending to 5	4	Minimum Recover

Week 4

Day 4 Lower Body

Exercise	Repetitions	Sets	Rest
Power Clean	7	5	1 minute
Hang Clean	7	5	1 minute
Snatch	7	5	1 minute
Back Squat	7	5	1 minute
Front Squat	7	5	1 minute
Military Press	7	5	1 minute
BB Abs Crunch/Leg Lift	20 Superset	3	Full Recovery

Week 5

Day 1 Upper Body

Exercise	Repetitions	Sets	Rest
Flat Bench BB	8	5	1 minute
Incline bench BB	8	5	1 minute
Clap Pushup	8	5	1 minute
Pushup	Max	3	Full Recovery
BB Row	8	5	1 minute
Pull Up	8	3	1 minute
Inverted Row	Max	3	Full Recovery
Pyramid Abs Crunch/Leg Lift/V Up	20 descending to 5	4	Minimum Recovery

Week 5

Day 2 Lower Body

Exercise	Repetitions	Sets	Rest
Power Clean	8	5	1 minute
Hang Clean	8	5	1 minute
Snatch	8	5	1 minute
Back Squat	8	5	1 minute
Front Squat	8	5	1 minute
Military Press	8	5	1 minute
BB Abs Crunch/Leg Lift	20 Superset	3	Full Recovery

Week 5

Day 3 Upper Body

Exercise	Repetitions	Sets	Rest
Flat Bench BB	8	5	1 minute
Incline bench BB	8	5	1 minute
Clap Pushup	8	5	1 minute
Pushup	Max	3	Full Recovery
BB Row	8	5	1 minute
Pull Up	8	3	1 minute
Inverted Row	Max	3	Full Recovery
Pyramid Abs Crunch/Leg Lift/V Up	20 descending to 5	4	Minimum Recover

Week 5

Day 4 Lower Body

Exercise	Repetitions	Sets	Rest
Power Clean	8	5	1 minute
Hang Clean	8	5	1 minute
Snatch	8	5	1 minute
Back Squat	8	5	1 minute
Front Squat	8	5	1 minute
Military Press	8	5	1 minute
BB Abs Crunch/Leg Lift	20 Superset	3	Full Recovery

Week 6

Day 1 Upper Body

Exercise	Repetitions	Sets	Rest
Flat Bench BB	6	5	1 minute
Incline bench BB	6	5	1 minute
Clap Pushup	6	5	1 minute
Pushup	Max	3	Full Recovery
BB Row	6	5	1 minute
Pull Up	6	3	1 minute
Inverted Row	Max	3	Full Recovery
Pyramid Abs Crunch/Leg Lift/V Up	20 descending to 5	4	Minimum Recovery

Week 6

Day 2 Lower Body

Exercise	Repetitions	Sets	Rest
Power Clean	6	5	1 minute
Hang Clean	6	5	1 minute
Snatch	6	5	1 minute
Back Squat	6	5	1 minute
Front Squat	6	5	1 minute
Military Press	6	5	1 minute
BB Abs Crunch/Leg Lift	20 Superset	3	Full Recovery

Week 6

Day 3 Upper Body

Exercise	Repetitions	Sets	Rest
Flat Bench BB	6	5	1 minute
Incline bench BB	6	5	1 minute
Clap Pushup	6	5	1 minute
Pushup	Max	3	Full Recovery
BB Row	6	5	1 minute
Pull Up	6	3	1 minute
Inverted Row	Max	3	Full Recovery
Pyramid Abs Crunch/Leg Lift/V Up	20 descending to 5	4	Minimum Recover

Week 6

Day 4 Lower Body

Exercise	Repetitions	Sets	Rest
Power Clean	6	5	1 minute
Hang Clean	6	5	1 minute
Snatch	6	5	1 minute
Back Squat	6	5	1 minute
Front Squat	6	5	1 minute
Military Press	6	5	1 minute
BB Abs Crunch/Leg Lift	20 Superset	3	Full Recovery

Week 7

Day 1 Upper Body

Exercise	Repetitions	Sets	Rest
Flat Bench BB	5	5	1 minute
Incline bench BB	5	5	1 minute
Clap Pushup	5	5	1 minute
Pushup	Max	3	Full Recovery
BB Row	5	5	1 minute
Pull Up	5	3	1 minute
Inverted Row	Max	3	Full Recovery
Pyramid Abs Crunch/Leg Lift/V Up	20 descending to 5	4	Minimum Recovery

Week 7

Day 2 Lower Body

Exercise	Repetitions	Sets	Rest
Power Clean	5	5	1 minute
Hang Clean	5	5	1 minute
Snatch	5	5	1 minute
Back Squat	5	5	1 minute
Front Squat	5	5	1 minute
Military Press	5	5	1 minute
BB Abs Crunch/Leg Lift	20 Superset	3	Full Recovery

Week 7

Day 3 Upper Body

Exercise	Repetitions	Sets	Rest
Flat Bench BB	5	5	1 minute
Incline bench BB	5	5	1 minute
Clap Pushup	5	5	1 minute
Pushup	Max	3	Full Recovery
BB Row	5	5	1 minute
Pull Up	5	3	1 minute
Inverted Row	Max	3	Full Recovery
Pyramid Abs Crunch/Leg Lift/V Up	20 descending to 5	4	Minimum Recover

Week 7

Day 4 Lower Body

Exercise	Repetitions	Sets	Rest
Power Clean	5	5	1 minute
Hang Clean	5	5	1 minute
Snatch	5	5	1 minute
Back Squat	5	5	1 minute
Front Squat	5	5	1 minute
Military Press	5	5	1 minute
BB Abs Crunch/Leg Lift	20 Superset	3	Full Recovery

Basic Body Balance/Active Recovery Cardio

Weeks 8-9

Refer to Cardio Schedule on Page 34

			Basic Body Balance Week 8					
	Day 1			**Day 2**			**Day 3**	
	Circuit 1			**Circuit 1**			**Circuit 1**	
	Exercise	**Reps**		**Exercise**	**Reps**		**Exercise**	**Reps**
1	Med Ball Pushups	10-15	1	One Leg Straight Leg Deadlift	10-15	1	One Arm Seated Chest Press	10-15
2	Pull Start	10-15	2	Bench Dip	10-15	2	One Legged Leg Press	10-15
3	One Leg Shoulder Press	10-15	3	Cable Chop Up	10-15	3	Cable Chop Down	10-15
	Circuit 2			**Circuit 2**			**Circuit 2**	
4	Cable Chop Up	10-15	4	One Legged Leg Press	10-15	4	One Arm Cable Row Standing	10-15
5	One Arm Lat Pulldown	10-15	5	One Leg triceps Pushdown	10-15	5	Med Ball Toss Lying On Back	10-15
6	Split Squat Rotating Cable P	10-15	6	Cable Chop Down	10-15	6	One Arm Alt Shoulder Press	10-15
	Circuit 3			**Circuit 3**			**Circuit 3**	
7	Med Ball Toss Lying	10-15	7	Squat and Rotate	10-15	7	Cable Chop Up	10-15
8	One Leg Inverted Row DB	10-15	8	Standing Triceps Kickback	10-15	8	Squat and Rotate	10-15
9	One Arm Shoulder Press	10-15	9	One Leg Hammer Curl	10-15	9	Dips Bench	10-15
	Abdominals			**Abdominals**			**Abdominals**	
	3 Supersets			**3 Supersets**			**3 Supersets**	
	Planks Front/Side/Back	3/30 Sec		Ball Crunch	20-30		Hanging Knee Raises	30
	Pull Down Cable Crunch	3/30		Windmills	20-30		Kneel Cable Crunch	30

Basic Body Balance Week 8

Day 1

	Circuit 1	
	Exercise	**Reps**
1	Med Ball Toss Lying	10-15
2	One Leg Inverted Row DB	10-15
3	One Arm Shoulder Press	10-15
	Circuit 2	
4	Med Ball Pushups	10-15
5	Pull Start	10-15
6	Cable Chop Up	10-15
	Circuit 3	
7	Alt Arm DB Inc	10-15
8	One Arm Lat Pulldown	10-15
9	Cable Chop Down	10-15
	Abdominals	
	3 Supersets	
	Pull Down Cable Crunch	3/40
	Planks Front/Side/Back	3/45 Sec

Day 2

	Circuit 1	
	Exercise	**Reps**
1	Squat and Rotate	10-15
2	Standing Triceps Kickback	10-15
3	One Leg Hammer Curl	10-15
	Circuit 2	
4	One Leg Straight Leg Dead Lift	10-15
5	Bench Dip	10-15
6	Cable Chop Up	10-15
	Circuit 3	
7	One Legged Leg Press	10-15
8	Cable Chop Down	10-15
9	One Leg DB Curl Twist	10-15
	Abdominals	
	3 Supersets	
	Windmills	20-30
	Ball Crunch	20-30

Day 3

	Circuit 1	
	Exercise	**Re**
1	Cable Chop Up	10
2	Squat and Rotate	10
3	Dips Bench	10
	Circuit 2	
4	One Arm Seated Chest Press	10
5	One Leg Leg Press	10
6	Cable Chop Down	10
	Circuit 3	
7	One Arm Cable Row Standing	1
8	Med Ball Toss Lying On Back	1
9	One Arm Alt Shoulder Press	1
	Abdominals	
	3 Supersets	
	Kneel Cable Crunch	
	Hanging Knee Raises	

Advanced Strength/Power

Weeks 10-14

Week 10

Day 1 Upper Body

Exercise	Repetitions	Sets	Rest
Flat Bench BB	6	5	1 minute
Incline Bench BB	6	5	1 minute
Flat Bench DB	6	5	1 minute
Lat Pulldown	6	5	1 minute
DB/BB Row	6	5	1 minute
Pull Ups	Max	4	Full Recovery
Push Up	Max	4	Full Recovery
Pyramid Abs Crunch/Leg Lift/V Up	25 descending to 10	4	Minimum Recovery

Week 10

Day 2 Lower Body

Execise	Repetitions	Sets	Rest
Back Squat	6	5	1 minute
Power Clean	6	5	1 minute
Hang Clean DB/BB	6	3 each	1 minute
Snatch DB/BB	3/6	3 each	1 minute
Front Squat	6	5	1 minute
Military Press	6	5	1 minute
BB Abs Crunches/Leg Lifts	20/Superset	3	Full Recovery

Week 10

Day 3 **Upper Body**

Exercise	Repetitions	Sets	Rest
Flat Bench BB	6	5	1 minute
Incline Bench BB	6	5	1 minute
Flat Bench DB	6	5	1 minute
Lat Pulldown	6	5	1 minute
DB/BB Row	6	5	1 minute
Pull Ups	Max	4	Full Recovery
Push Up	Max	4	Full Recovery
Pyramid Abs Crunch/Leg Lift/V Up	25 descending to 10	4	Minimum Recovery

Week 10

Day 4 **Lower Body**

Execise	Repetitions	Sets	Rest
Back Squat	7	5	1 minute
Power Clean	7	5	1 minute
Hang Clean DB/BB	7	3 each	1 minute
Snatch DB/BB	3/7	3 each	1 minute
Front Squat	7	5	1 minute
Military Press	7	5	1 minute
BB Abs Crunches/Leg Lifts	20/Superset	3	Full Recovery

Week 11

Day 1 Upper Body

Exercise	Repetitions	Sets	Rest
Flat Bench BB	7	5	1 minute
Incline Bench BB	7	5	1 minute
Flat Bench DB	7	5	1 minute
Lat Pulldown	7	5	1 minute
DB/BB Row	7	5	1 minute
Pull Ups	Max	4	Full Recovery
Push Up	Max	4	Full Recovery
Pyramid Abs Crunch/Leg Lift/V Up	25 descending to 10	4	Minimum Recovery

Week 11

Day 2 Lower Body

Execise	Repetitions	Sets	Rest
Back Squat	7	5	1 minute
Power Clean	7	5	1 minute
Hang Clean DB/BB	7	3 each	1 minute
Snatch DB/BB	3/7	3 each	1 minute
Front Squat	7	5	1 minute
Military Press	7	5	1 minute
BB Abs Crunches/Leg Lifts	20/Superset	3	Full Recovery

Week 11

Day 3 **Upper Body**

Exercise	Repetitions	Sets	Rest
Flat Bench BB	7	5	1 minute
Incline Bench BB	7	5	1 minute
Flat Bench DB	7	5	1 minute
Lat Pulldown	7	5	1 minute
DB/BB Row	7	5	1 minute
Pull Ups	Max	4	Full Recovery
Push Up	Max	4	Full Recovery
Pyramid Abs Crunch/Leg Lift/V Up	25 descending to 10	4	Minimum Recovery

Week 11

Day 4 **Lower Body**

Execise	Repetitions	Sets	Rest
Back Squat	7	5	1 minute
Power Clean	7	5	1 minute
Hang Clean DB/BB	7	3 each	1 minute
Snatch DB/BB	3/7	3 each	1 minute
Front Squat	7	5	1 minute
Military Press	7	5	1 minute
BB Abs Crunches/Leg Lifts	20/Superset	3	Full Recovery

Week 12

Day 1 Upper Body

Exercise	Repetitions	Sets	Rest
Flat Bench BB	8	5	1 minute
Incline Bench BB	8	5	1 minute
Flat Bench DB	8	5	1 minute
Lat Pulldown	8	5	1 minute
DB/BB Row	8	5	1 minute
Pull Ups	Max	4	Full Recovery
Push Up	Max	4	Full Recovery
Pyramid Abs Crunch/Leg Lift/V Up	25 descending to 10	4	Minimum Recovery

Week 12

Day 2 Lower Body

Execise	Repetitions	Sets	Rest
Back Squat	8	5	1 minute
Power Clean	8	5	1 minute
Hang Clean DB/BB	8	3 each	1 minute
Snatch DB/BB	4/8	3 each	1 minute
Front Squat	8	5	1 minute
Military Press	8	5	1 minute
BB Abs Crunches/Leg Lifts	20/Superset	3	Full Recovery

Week 12

Day 3 Upper Body

Exercise	Repetitions	Sets	Rest
Flat Bench BB	8	5	1 minute
Incline Bench BB	8	5	1 minute
Flat Bench DB	8	5	1 minute
Lat Pulldown	8	5	1 minute
DB/BB Row	8	5	1 minute
Pull Ups	Max	4	Full Recovery
Push Up	Max	4	Full Recovery
Pyramid Abs Crunch/Leg Lift/V Up	25 descending to 10	4	Minimum Recovery

Week 12

Day 4 Lower Body

Execise	Repetitions	Sets	Rest
Back Squat	8	5	1 minute
Power Clean	8	5	1 minute
Hang Clean DB/BB	8	3 each	1 minute
Snatch DB/BB	4/8	3 each	1 minute
Front Squat	8	5	1 minute
Military Press	8	5	1 minute
BB Abs Crunches/Leg Lifts	20/Superset	3	Full Recovery

Week 13

Day 1 Upper Body

Exercise	Repetitions	Sets	Rest
Flat Bench BB	8	5	1 minute
Incline Bench BB	8	5	1 minute
Flat Bench DB	8	5	1 minute
Lat Pulldown	8	5	1 minute
DB/BB Row	8	5	1 minute
Pull Ups	Max	4	Full Recovery
Push Up	Max	4	Full Recovery
Pyramid Abs Crunch/Leg Lift/V Up	25 descending to 10	4	Minimum Recovery

Week 13

Day 2 Lower Body

Execise	Repetitions	Sets	Rest
Back Squat	8	5	1 minute
Power Clean	8	5	1 minute
Hang Clean DB/BB	8	3 each	1 minute
Snatch DB/BB	4/8	3 each	1 minute
Front Squat	8	5	1 minute
Military Press	8	5	1 minute
BB Abs Crunches/Leg Lifts	20/Superset	3	Full Recovery

Week 13

Day 3 Upper Body

Exercise	Repetitions	Sets	Rest
Flat Bench BB	8	5	1 minute
Incline Bench BB	8	5	1 minute
Flat Bench DB	8	5	1 minute
Lat Pulldown	8	5	1 minute
DB/BB Row	8	5	1 minute
Pull Ups	Max	4	Full Recovery
Push Up	Max	4	Full Recovery
Pyramid Abs Crunch/Leg Lift/V Up	25 descending to 10	4	Minimum Recovery

Week 13

Day 4 Lower Body

Execise	Repetitions	Sets	Rest
Back Squat	8	5	1 minute
Power Clean	8	5	1 minute
Hang Clean DB/BB	8	3 each	1 minute
Snatch DB/BB	4/8	3 each	1 minute
Front Squat	8	5	1 minute
Military Press	8	5	1 minute
BB Abs Crunches/Leg Lifts	20/Superset	3	Full Recovery

Week 14

Day 1 Upper Body

Exercise	Repetitions	Sets	Rest
Flat Bench BB	5	5	1 minute
Incline Bench BB	5	5	1 minute
Flat Bench DB	5	5	1 minute
Lat Pulldown	5	5	1 minute
DB/BB Row	5	5	1 minute
Pull Ups	Max	4	Full Recovery
Push Up	Max	4	Full Recovery
Pyramid Abs Crunch/Leg Lift/V Up	25 descending to 10	4	Minimum Recovery

Week 14

Day 2 Lower Body

Execise	Repetitions	Sets	Rest
Back Squat	5	5	1 minute
Power Clean	5	5	1 minute
Hang Clean DB/BB	5	3 each	1 minute
Snatch DB/BB	3/5	3 each	1 minute
Front Squat	5	5	1 minute
Military Press	5	5	1 minute
BB Abs Crunches/Leg Lifts	20/Superset	3	Full Recovery

Week 14

Day 3 Upper Body

Exercise	Repetitions	Sets	Rest
Flat Bench BB	5	5	1 minute
Incline Bench BB	5	5	1 minute
Flat Bench DB	5	5	1 minute
Lat Pulldown	5	5	1 minute
DB/BB Row	5	5	1 minute
Pull Ups	Max	4	Full Recovery
Push Up	Max	4	Full Recovery
Pyramid Abs Crunch/Leg Lift/V Up	25 descending to 10	4	Minimum Recovery

Week 14

Day 4 Lower Body

Execise	Repetitions	Sets	Rest
Back Squat	5	5	1 minute
Power Clean	5	5	1 minute
Hang Clean DB/BB	5	3 each	1 minute
Snatch DB/BB	3/5	3 each	1 minute
Front Squat	5	5	1 minute
Military Press	5	5	1 minute
BB Abs Crunches/Leg Lifts	20/Superset	3	Full Recovery

Advanced Body Balance/Active Recovery Cardio

Weeks 15-16

Refer to Cardio Schedule on page 34

Advanced Body Balance
Week 15

Day 1

Circuit 1

	Exercise	Reps
1a	Alt Bench DB	10-15
1b	One Arm Seated Chest Press	10-15
2a	DB One Leg Bent Row	10-15
2b	Pull Start	10-15
3a	One Leg Shoulder Press DB	10-15
3b	Shoulder Press Diff Lbs	10-15

Circuit 2

	Exercise	Reps
4a	One Arm DB Inc	10-15
4b	Med Ball Pushups	10-15
5a	Pull Ups	10-15
5b	One Arm Lat Pulldown	10-15
6a	One Leg Upright Row w/ Cable	10-15
6b	Split Squat Rotating Cable Row	10-15

Circuit 3

	Exercise	Reps
7a	Hand Walks	10-15
7b	Med Ball Toss Lying	10-15
8a	One Leg Inverted Row DB	10-15
8b	One Leg Inverted Row Cable	10-15
9a	One Arm Alt Shoulder Press	10-15

Day2

Circuit 1

	Exercise	Reps
1a	One Leg Deadlift	10-15
1b	One Leg Hamstring Curl	10-15
2a	Dips Roman Chair	10-15
2b	Dips Bench	10-15
3a	Bicep Cable Curl	10-15
3b	Bicep Curl BB	10-15

Circuit 2

	Exercise	Reps
4a	One Leg Squats	10-15
4b	One Leg Extension	10-15
5a	One Leg Tri Pushdowns	10-15
5b	Overhead Tri Ext	10-15
6a	One Leg DB Curl Alt	10-15
6b	One Leg Cable Curls	10-15

Circuit 3

	Exercise	Reps
7a	Squat and Rotate	10-15
7b	Lunge and Rotate	10-15
8a	One Leg Standing Tri Kickback	10-15
8b	Tri Overhead Ext	10-15
9a	One Leg Hammer Curl	10-15

Day 3

Circuit 1

	Exercise	Rep
1a	One Arm Seated Chest Press	10-
1b	Med Ball Pushups	10-
2a	One Leg Hamstring Curl	10-
2b	One Leg Hyperextension	10-
3a	Cable Chop Down	10-
3b	One Leg Straight Arm Pull	10-

Circuit 2

	Exercise	Rep
4a	One Leg Inverted Row	10-
4b	One Arm Cable Row Standing	10-
5a	Hand Walks	10-
5b	Med Ball Toss Lying on Back	10-
6a	One Arm Alt Shoulder Press	10-
6b	One Leg DB Shoulder Press	10-

Circuit 3

	Exercise	Rep
7a	Lunge & Rotate	10
7b	Squat & Rotate	10
8a	Dips Bench	10
8b	Dips Roman Chair	10
9a	Cable Chop Up	10

9b	One Leg DB Shoulder Press	10-15
Abdominals		
3 Supersets		
Planks Front/Side/Back		3/30 sec
Pull Down Cable Crunch		3/20

9b	One Leg Alt Curl	10-15
Abdominals		
3 Supersets		
Ball Crunch		15-20
Windmills		15-20

9b	Trunk Rotations Cable	10-15
Abdominals		
3 Supersets		
Hanging Knee Raises		20
Kneel Cable Crunch		20

Advanced Body Balance
Week 16

Day 1		
Circuit 1		
	Exercise	**Reps**
1a	One Arm Seated Chest Press	10-15
1b	One Arm Bench DB	10-15
2a	Pull Start	10-15
2b	One Leg Bent Row DB	10-15
3a	Shoulder Press Diff Lbs	10-15
3b	One Leg Shoulder Press DB	10-15
Circuit 2		
4a	Med Ball Pushups	10-15
4b	One Arm DB Inc	10-15
5a	One Arm Lat Pulldown	10-15
5b	Pull Ups	10-15
6a	Split Squat Rotating Cable Row	10-15
6b	One Leg Upright Row w/ Cable	10-15
Circuit 3		
7a	Med Ball Toss Lying	10-15
7b	Hand Walks	10-15
8a	One Leg Inverted Row Cable	10-15
8b	One Leg Inverted Row DB	10-15
9a	One Leg DB Shoulder Press	10-15

Day 2		
Circuit 1		
	Exercise	**Reps**
1a	One Leg Hamstring Curl	10-15
1b	One Leg Deadlift	10-15
2a	Dips Bench	10-15
2b	Dips Roman Chair	10-15
3a	Bicep Curl BB	10-15
3b	Bicep Cable Curl	10-15
Circuit 2		
4a	One Leg Extension	10-15
4b	One Leg Squats	10-15
5a	Overhead Tri Ext	10-15
5b	One Leg Tri Pushdowns	10-15
6a	One Leg Cable Curls	10-15
6b	One Leg DB Curl Alt	10-15
Circuit 3		
7a	Lunge and Rotate	10-15
7b	Squat and Rotate	10-15
8a	Tri Overhead Ext	10-15
8b	One Leg Standing Tri Kickbakcs	10-15
9a	One Leg Bicep Curl	10-15

Day 3		
Circuit 1		
	Exercise	**Re**
1a	Med Ball Pushups	10
1b	One Arm Seated Chest Press	10
2a	One Leg Hyperextensions	10
2b	One Leg Hamstring Curll	10
3a	One Arm Straight Arm Pull	10
3b	Cable Chop Down	10
Circuit 2		
4a	One Arm Cable Row Standing	10
4b	One Leg Inverted Row	1
5a	Med Ball Toss Lying On Back	1
5b	Hand Walks	1
6a	One Leg DB Shoulder Press	1
6b	One Arm Alt Shoulder Press	1
Circuit 3		
7a	Squat and Rotate	1
7b	Lunge and Rotate	1
8a	Dips Roman Chair	1
8b	Dips Bench	1
9a	Trunk Rotations Cable	1

9b	One Arm Alt Shoulder Press	10-15
Abdominals		
3 Supersets		
Pull Down Cable Crunch		3/30 sec
Planks Front/Side/Back		3/20

9b	One Leg Hammer Curl	10-15
Abdominals		
3 Supersets		
Windmills		15-20
Ball Crunch		15-20

9b	Cable Chop Up	10-15
Abdominals		
3 Supersets		
Kneel Cable Crunch		20
Hanging Knee Raises		20

www.ingramcontent.com/pod-product-compliance
Ingram Content Group UK Ltd.
Pitfield, Milton Keynes, MK11 3LW, UK
UKHW020138250726
13967UKWH00002B/727

9 781678 183141